Pain: Causes and Treatment of Pain Associated with Fibromyalgia, Arthritis and Soft Tissue Injury

By
Lynne D M Noble

Copyright 2018 Lynne D M Noble

Independently published

Contents

Dedication

This book is dedicated to all who suffer joint and rheumatic pain

Acknowledgement

Many thanks to all my friends who have supplied the inspiration to write this book.

Preface

There is no doubt that thousands of working hours are lost every year due to chronic or acute pain of the joints and surrounding tissues. Studies suggest that forty-nine out of every people will suffer from this type of pain in their lives so the impact on the quality of life is enormous.

There are over 220 different types of rheumatic disease and they are divided into four main groups.   These are the non-inflammatory osteoarthritis, the inflammatory arthritis, back pain and soft tissue rheumatism.

In some cases, joint may become progressively damaged and need replacing at some point if they are not to cause serious disability. In other cases, symptoms may be relatively mild. They may cause some background pain but little disability. In some cases, the discomfort may disappear entirely.

Medication is used to treat the symptoms in all four of the above categories although it is not a cure. They can reduce pain to more manageable levels and slow progression.

What of those individuals whose pain cannot be controlled? This could be due to the fact that their pain is too severe yet they have had their daily quota of painkillers or they cannot take conventional painkillers. Non-steroidal anti-inflammatory drugs (NSAID's) such as ibuprofen can cause severe allergic shock in some people. Individuals on methotrexate which is a disease modifying drug, cannot take NSAID's. Their choice of analgesia is limited.

When circumstances limit the type and amount of painkillers we can take, then we have to look towards alternative solutions. There are indeed a great many but they are not part of popular knowledge. As they are easily obtainable it does not pay the pharmaceutical companies to market them since they would not create profit for industry.

This book is intended to help the reader understand the underlying causes of pain in some of the most prevalent joint and soft tissue condition and, just as importantly what can be done about it.

An Overview of Joint Pain

Joint pain will affect just about everyone at some point in their life. The medical term of joint pain is arthralgia and when it is accompanied by joint inflammation then it is referred to as arthritis. Inflammation causes serious pain and swelling. Inflamed joints may also be warm and red. Other symptoms may accompany these signs of inflammation depending on the underlying cause. These may include symptoms such as a fever, mouth sores or rash, among others.

The normal joint consists of the place where two ends of bones meet. At the ends of these bones is a smooth layer of cartilage which acts as a shock absorber. The cartilage is often referred to as 'gristle.'

Surrounding the bones there is a membrane called the synovial membrane. This produces a sticky fluid called synovial fluid. This helps to nourish and lubricate the cartilage. The ligaments surround the synovial membrane. They are thick broad bands which help to keep the joint stable and stop it moving beyond a normal range. Tendons can be found outside the ligaments and help attach muscles to bone.

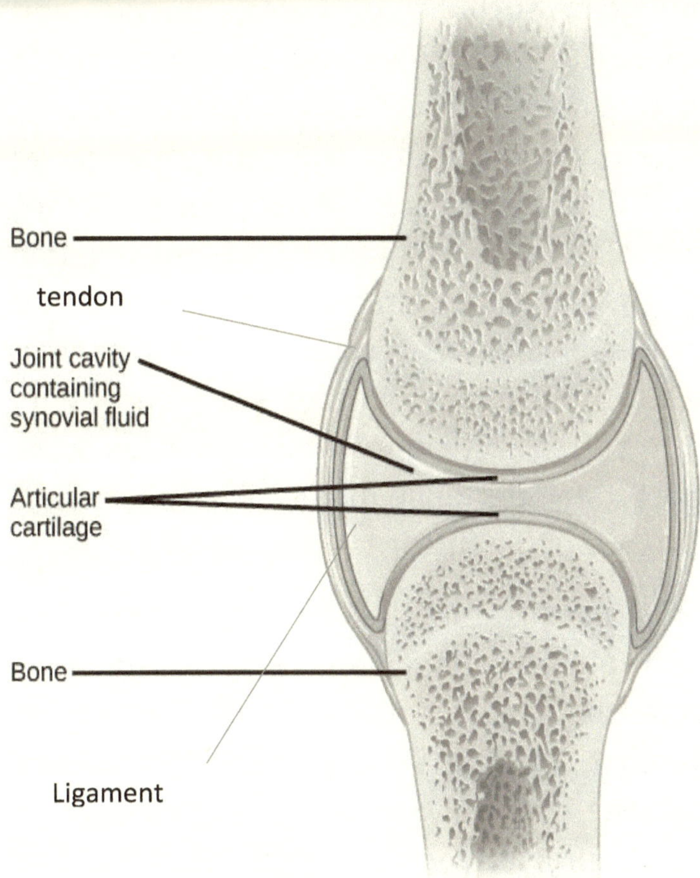

1.   A typical joint

Not all pain which appears to be radiating from joints is actually joint pain. It is not unusual for pain to be coming from structures close to the painful joint such as ligaments, muscles and tendons. The latter conditions seem to occur in those who are quite active and whose joints may be hypermobile so that the joint may move beyond a normal range. Many people are not aware of the hypermobility of their joints although, if they look back, they may realise that they probably had more sprains and strains than others around them. As they get older, joints tend to stiffen somewhat which provides more support to hypermobile joints. As such there is less chance of damaging connective tissue.

When true arthralgia does occur then the pattern of joint pain can vary according to whether the joint is rested or in use. Sometimes a number of joints may be affected and sometimes it is only one. When a number of joints are affected then there you often find that the corresponding joint is also affected. Generally, this appears to be the joints of the hands and knees but there are variations.

There is also a condition known as migratory arthritis which appears to flit about from joint to joint. Once I presented at my GP with a very inflamed swollen left ankle for which there had been no obvious injury. I was referred to rheumatology and by the time my appointment came around to see the consultant, the swelling in my left ankle had disappeared. However, my right ankle was pumped up like a balloon and was hot and tender.

There are many causes of arthritis. There may be a flare up of a chronic existing auto-immune disorder such as rheumatoid arthritis. These acute flare ups generally affect many joints and can make the patient feel quite poorly. However, other causes include viruses, Lyme disease, streptococcal bacterial infections, gout and reactive arthritis. Reactive arthritis is a type of arthritis that develops after an infection – generally of the urinary or digestive tract.

 Chronic arthritis which affects multiple joints is most likely to be due to the inflammatory disorders such as Systemic Lupus Erythematosis, rheumatoid or psoriatic arthritis. There is also a non-inflammatory disorder known as osteoarthritis. This is rife and by the time middle age arrives most people appear to have some osteoarthritis in one or more of their joints. These tend to be the hips or knees due to their load bearing capacity. This is the reason why adults are cautioned to lose weight if they have osteoarthritis.

The most common pain which radiates external to the joint are:

- Fibromyalgia
- Polymyalgia rheumatica
- Tendonitis or bursitis

In the case of fibromyalgia, the cause is not known. However, fibromyalgia shares its symptoms with the damage and pain wreaked by an oft overlooked inflammatory mediator. We shall explore this in more detail later.

Tendonitis and bursitis are quite common in the population. Tendonitis can take a long time to heal and is very painful – as it bursitis. We will explore ways of reducing the time taken to heal and how we can reduce the level of pain until the injury has healed. Firstly, though, we need to look at inflammation and how it contributes to symptoms of pain, redness and swelling. Pain will then begin to make sense and you will have the beginnings of control over it.

What is inflammation?

Inflammation is a localised physical condition in which part of the body becomes reddened, swollen, hot and often painful, especially as a reaction to injury or infection.

Inflammation is a response to the damage done to living tissues through injury or infection. It is a defence mechanism designed to

- Localise the cause
- Eliminate it
- Remove the damaged tissue so than healing can begin

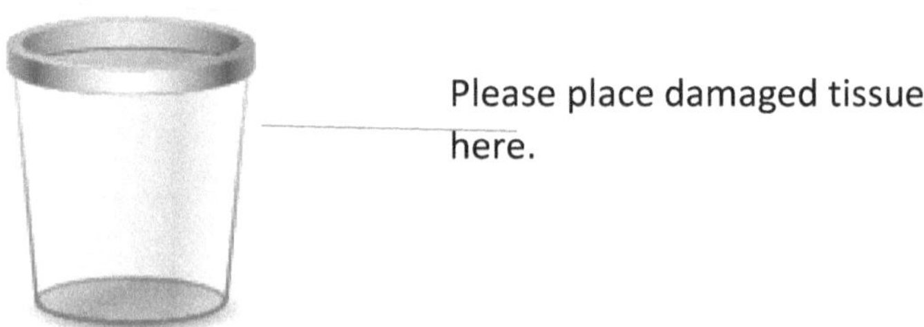

At the beginning of this process, the blood vessels become leaky. This allows fluid, protein

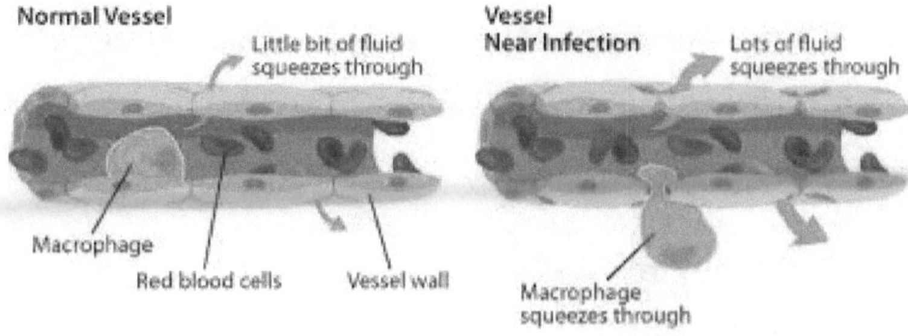

1

and white blood cells to move from the blood vessels into the site of the injury.

If this process only lasts a few days, then it is referred to as acute inflammation. If it lasts for much longer then it is referred to as chronic inflammation.

We need acute inflammation to provide the means for repair such as materials like protein and white blood cells which either destroy the infection or 'eat up' the damaged tissue before carting it away.

------

[1] https://askabiologist.asu.edu/macrophage

Following the release of the white blood cells a number of different substances are liberated.

Some of these substances are

- Bradykinin
- Serotonin
- Prostaglandins
- Histamine
- Substance P

This process generally brings along a number of unpleasant symptoms. These include

- Pain
- Itching
- Swelling (which limits movement and presses on nerves increasing pain).

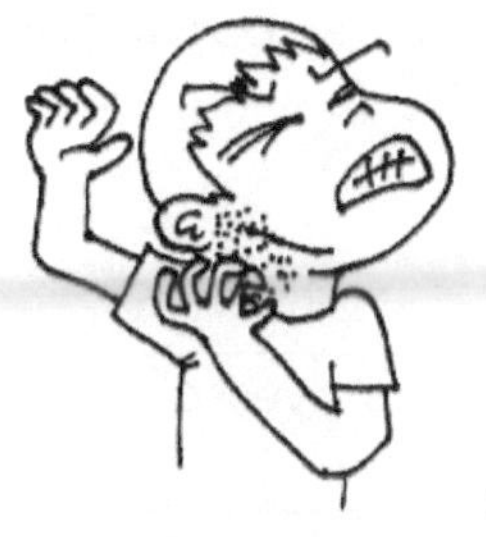

When white cells are liberated they release a number of chemicals. These can cause itching pain and swelling.

When healing has taken place the inflammatory process is no longer needed. However, sometimes it gets out of control. The inflammatory response doesn't work properly. It continues when it shouldn't. It begins to attack healthy tissue since all the damaged tissue has already been cleared away. This is what happens in auto-immune diseases such as rheumatoid arthritis.

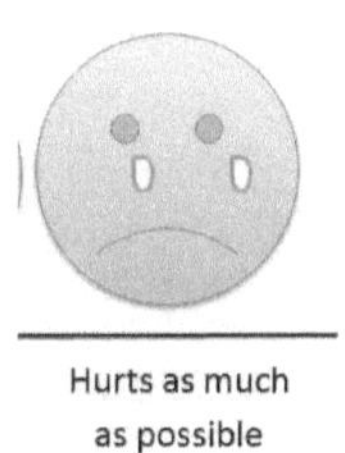

Hurts as much
as possible

---

[2] http://clipart-library.com/clipart/18585.htm

Table showing some important substances involved in pain

Bradykinin	Causes blood vessels to dilate
Serotonin	The brain uses serotonin to perpetuate chronic pain signals in local nerves. They also cause pain in undamaged areas adjacent to damaged areas of tissue
Prostaglandins	High levels of prostaglandins are produced in response to injury or infection and cause inflammation. They are associated with the symptoms of pain, redness, fever and swelling.
Histamine	Released from mast cells it causes widespread pain and many other symptoms
Substance P	Released from many immune system cells and is involved in chronic pain especially joint pain

Sometimes the inflammatory response is not strong enough to clear away infection or damaged tissue. This often happens with those individuals who have impaired immune systems due to advanced age, long term illness or poor nutrition, among others. At such times, wounds may fester and advance. The prescribing of antibiotics will be the correct response. However, it is also preferable if the immune system is kept in tip top condition as this will help to avoid the above scenario. Keeping the immune system in good working order   is achieved by getting sufficient rest, a good, varied diet and some exercise.

 Getting enough vitamin D through the action of the sunlight on the skin and in diet is vital. Vitamin D is needed for the production of antimicrobials which are antibacterial, antiviral and antifungal. Vitamin D is one of the unsung heroes of the vitamin world. When people think about vitamin D − if they do at all - they think of it in association with healthy bones. Most people do not realise that vitamin D makes its own antimicrobial called cathelicidin. Further, as the majority of the world are vitamin D deficient, this suggests that the majority of the world aren't harnessing the power within their own immune systems.

An antimicrobial, like cathelicidin, is an agent that kills microorganisms or stops their growth.

Cathelicidins are small antimicrobial peptides. They are part of our innate immune system and show a broad spectrum of antimicrobial activity against

- Bacteria
- Enveloped viruses
- Fungi

As well as exerting direct antimicrobial effects such as punching holes in the cell membranes of invaders, the cathelicidins can also trigger specific defence responses in the host.

Vitamin D upregulates the production of cathelicidins and is found to exert an effect in many organs and systems of the body. This is not surprising since vitamin D receptors can be found throughout the body.

Cathelicidins have been found in the:

- Stomach
- Trachea
- Skin
- Muscle
- Heart
- Kidney
- Lung
- Brain
- Intestine

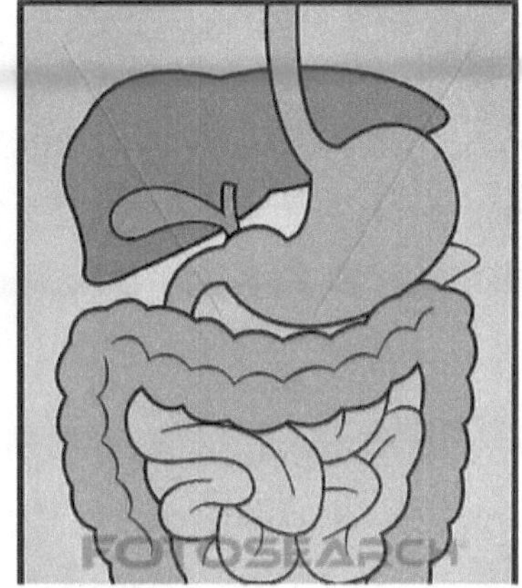

Cathelicidins have been found in the digestive system.

as well as joints.

Human cathelicidin acts in the promotion of wound healing and can modulate the adaptive immune system.

As people get older they are less likely to be able to absorb vitamin D through their skin. Older people and those with inflammatory bowel disease have greater difficulty absorbing any nutrient from food.   Further, it is extremely difficult, if not impossible, to obtain sufficient vitamin D from the diet.

The best sources of vitamin D are oily fish, fortified cereals and eggs. However, you would need to eat 80 eggs daily to obtain sufficient vitamin D for the day. The recommended daily amount is 1000-4000 IU's.

Intense exercise can actually impair the immune system. Even though this is only temporary, the exercise to be found in housework, gardening and walking to the shops is generally adequate.

A little light exercise is fine but too much can impair the immune system so that it cannot fight infection or remove damaged tissue.

Responses to chemicals, illness or injury causing pain

One of the questions that I get asked a lot is whether we should take any medication at times of illness or injury since the immune system is just doing its job.

Pain, in general, is debilitating and sometimes is felt out of all proportion to the injury or severity of the illness. The immune system has a tendency to throw everything it has when it is alerted to tissue damage, regardless of the reason. Any injury or illness is helped by a good night's rest so pain relief assists with this.

The recommendation for back pain is exercise. Back pain can be severe and is likely to be undertaken only with the assistance of pain relief. Although many medics believe that people with back pain should continue moving, acute pain is very painful. The understanding behind the 'keep moving' advice is that movement will mean that muscle mass will not be lost and further, movement will increase the movement of immune system cells to the site of injury to help with repair.

The latter can be accomplished by very gentle massage and the application of hot and cold packs.

Keeping muscles from atrophying will not be a problem for a couple of days and exercising does not mean going for a five mile walk. A small amount of stretching will be better than nothing for the early stages of back pain.

Whenever pain occurs, there is a corresponding pathway formed in the brain. At first the pathway is nebulous. It has the ability to fade provided pain does not continue. If pain does continue over a long time or is intense, even for a short time, then the pathway to pain becomes

1)   Pain pathway initially registered

2 Repeated or intense pain creates a default pain memory.

17

quite deeply etched. It becomes a default pathway where even the slightest stimulus will set it off. Pain relief, at the right time can help stop this process.

Antibiotics are a necessity when a bacterial infection is not being controlled by the immune system. This can occur for a number of reasons in susceptible groups such as

- Those with an underlying illness which has impaired the immune system
- Steroid and disease modifying drugs (DMARDS)[3] use.
- The elderly
- The young
- Those whose diet is not nutritionally sound
- Those who have another underlying condition which compromises the immune system

---

[3] Disease-modifying antirheumatic drugs (**DMARDs**) is a category of otherwise unrelated drugs defined by their use in rheumatoid arthritis to slow down disease progression.

Serotonin –

Serotonin is an important molecule in processing and modulating pin. It can cause pain as well as relieve it.

If serotonin acts in the peripheral nervous system then it makes pain worse in inflammation and nerve injury.

Chronic pain seems to cause serotonin to be released by the brain into the spinal cord. It acts on the trigeminal nerve which sets of processes which eventually leads to the nerves becoming even more excitable. Consequently, they send more pain signals to the brain.

It is easy to see how a pain memory can form.

There are a number of prescription drugs which alter serotonin levels. They are used to treat migraine, depression and nausea.

 Serotonin does not cross the blood brain barrier and therefore it has to be made inside the brain. Its precursor is tryptophan which is found in a number of foods such as

- Chocolate
- Chicken
- Eggs
- Milk
- Turkey
- Cheese
- Peanuts
- Fish
- Pumpkin and sesame seeds
- Tofu and soy

Light and exercise as well as the above high tryptophan foods enable the production of serotonin. Therefore, if chronic joint pain is a problem then reducing the amount of the tryptophan containing foods, reducing light levels and taking rest may help.

Bradykinins

Bradykinin can cause localised pain by increasing the permeability of blood vessels allowing materials necessary for repair and elimination to take place. The swelling that is caused will press on nerve endings increasing pain.

Some studies have found that bradykinin raises internal calcium levels in astrocytes (cells found in the brain). This causes a release of a substance called glutamate. Glutamate has been implicated in initiating pain.

There are a number of foods which inhibit bradykinins. Bromelain – found in pineapple – suppresses trauma induced swelling caused by the release of bradykinin into the bloodstream and then the tissues.

Red wine and polyphenols found in green tea and red wine also contain bradykinin inhibitors as does aloe.

Prostaglandins

These are substances which are produced by just about every tissue in the body. They generally act locally and are inactivated very readily.

Anti-inflammatories, like ibuprofen, act very well on prostaglandins. The difficulty is that anti-inflammatories have a number of unwanted side effects. Further, they are not suitable for

- those on DMARD's
- those with stomach ulcers
- peptic ulcer or stomach bleeding
- Uncontrolled hypertension
- People that suffer with inflammatory bowel disease
- Those with kidney disease
- Those with asthma
- Those who have had stroke

Among others.

Further unwanted side effects, found in various studies, are that NSAID's can delay muscle regeneration and slow the progress of ligament, tendon, muscle regeneration and cartilage healing.

Studies have found that NSAID's wipe out the entire inflammatory mediated flourish of white blood cells over 0-4 days which is required for healing.

Further studies showed that those who took NSAID's after an acute hamstring injury did not experience a greater reduction of pain and soft-tissue swelling compared with the placebo group.

It appeared that the NSAID's group had worse pain associated with severe injuries compared with the placebo group.

In order to avoid the potential difficulties of NSAID's, a number of natural substances can be substituted. These include

- Oily fish as research has shown that polyunsaturated fatty acids are some of the most effective natural anti-inflammatory substances there are.
- Curcumin is a yellow pigment made from turmeric and is used as a colouring and a flavouring. It has anti-inflammatory properties and is often used as an

effective substitute for people with joint inflammation.

The usual dose of turmeric powder would be 500mg three times daily.

- Green tea has anti-inflammatory and cartilage protective effects
- Grated fresh ginger also blocks the effects of prostaglandins

The foods to avoid as they increase inflammation are

- meat cooked at very high temperatures
- sunflower oil
- corn and corn oil
- soy beans
- fried foods
- processed snacks
- margarine

Histamine deserves a lot of examination. Its effects are systemic and so excessive histamine or an intolerance to histamine can make you feel very ill indeed.

Histamine is found in mast cells which are white cells of the immune system. The mast cells are generally located in nearby connective tissue. Histamine has a similar affect to prostaglandins. It has an important role in the early inflammatory response and therefore is associated more with acute inflammation.

As histamine's actions are not localised, they can cause widespread pain

While histamine is normally associated with acute inflammation, it is also associated with chronic inflammation. It regulates several vital roles in the immune response.

There is quite a widespread condition called histamine intolerance which is, nevertheless, little known about. It has a myriad of symptoms including

- pain associated with inflammation as can be found in rheumatic diseases or rheumatoid arthritis such as knuckle joint rheumatism.

- soft tissue rheumatism eg pain in the tendons, joints, back pain. Studies show that soft tissue rheumatism feels like a strained muscle or muscle ache.

The Marion institute stated that histamine could be responsible for muscular rheumatism or inflammation of a muscle.[4]as well as the above.

People with histamine intolerance tend to feel very ill, very often.

---

[4] https://www.marioninstitute.org/histamine-intolerance-syndrome/

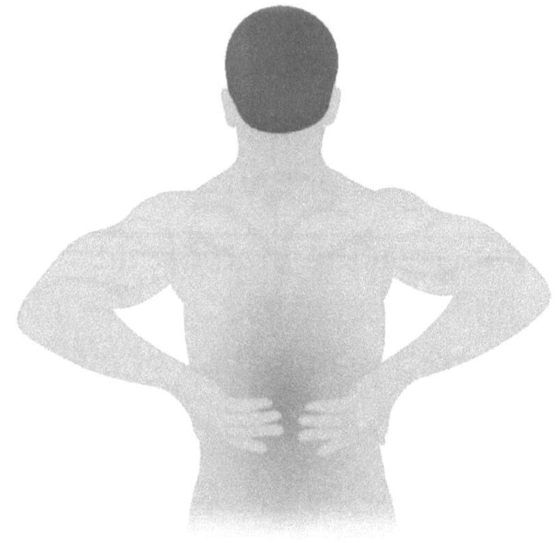

The effects are much more widespread than this, but these studies show that often muscle ache has nothing to do with any injury to the muscle. Histamine intolerance can make you feel truly awful.

The best way to counteract the effects of histamine intolerance is to go on a low histamine diet.

Histamine is found in many foods nowadays such as

- tomato ketchup
- fermented foods
- anything pickled
- cured or fermented meats
- wine beer alcohol
- tomatoes, aubergine, spinach
- canned fish

It is quite difficult to avoid foods containing histamine but fresh foods will contain less histamine than if they stored for a couple of days before being eaten.

Of course antihistamines are an effective treatment for histamine intolerance. Antihistamines work very well in many types of chronic pain which is entirely unrelated to the allergies which is often associated with. If you have joint pain it is well worth trying an antihistamine which have far fewer side effects than NSAID's.

Professor Theoharis Theorharides of Tufts University found that two drugs used in treating pain –amytriptyline and doxepin elixir – just happened to have histamine reducing properties.

Diamine oxidase (DAO) is the major enzyme involved in histamine metabolism. It ensures that there is the correct level of histamine available required for the balance of numerous chemical reactions taking place in the body.

DAO also degrades any extracellular (free) histamine which might have occurred through diet or from allergy induced processes in the body.

Olive oil has been found to release DAO into the bloodstream by up to 500%[5]

---

[5] Wollin, A, wang, X, Tso, P. (2017) Nutrients regulate diamine oxidase release from intestinal mucosa). The American Physiological Society, 20, 220

Vitamin C is well known for acting in an antihistamine like way. Blood histamine levels seem to be inversely associated with the amount of circulating vitamin C so that the greater the vitamin C the less histamine there will be.

Vitamin C, like vitamin B6, is a cofactor of DAO and so sufficient of these vitamins are required to make DAO. Vitamin C is found in fresh fruit and vegetables. It is easily destroyed by cooking. Vitamin B is found in meat, nuts and whole grains.

Zinc prevents the release of histamine from mast cells. It is found in

- Meat
- Fish, especially shellfish
- Dairy
- Eggs
- wholegrains

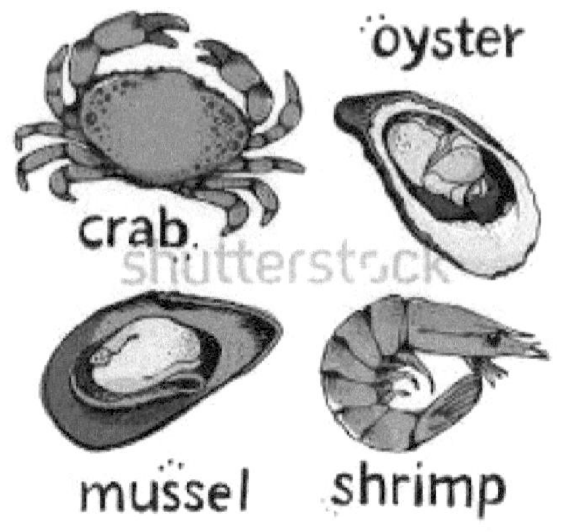

6

Shellfish contains lots of zinc which prevents release of histamine from mast cells.

but often, zinc supplementation is recommended when there is a histamine intolerance.

Substance P

Substance P is a transmitting chemical. It is released from the ends of specific sensory nerves

---

6 http://worldartsme.com/oysters-and-shrimp-clipart.html#gal_post_26674_oysters-and-shrimp-clipart-1.jpg

and is found in the central and peripheral nervous system. Therefore, its potential to cause pain is widespread.

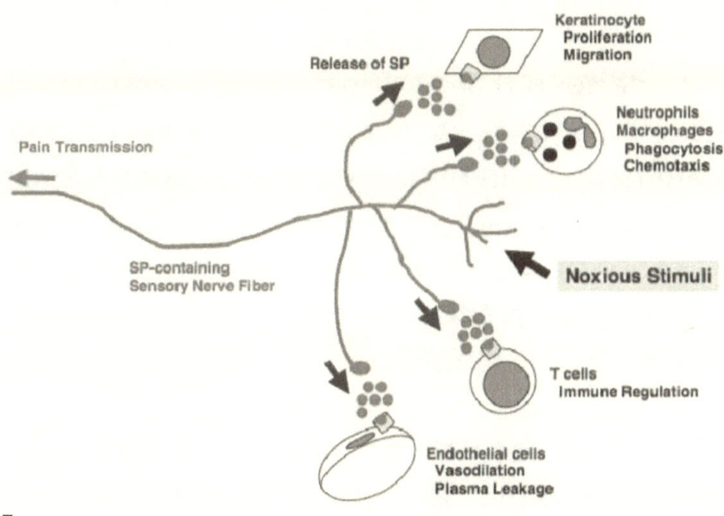

7

The nerve endings above come into contact with a noxious stimuli – chemical irritant, cold, heat etc and transfer it to a Substance P containing nerve fibre. Substance P is capable of transmitting pain (green arrow).
It can also bind to a wide variety of immune system cells and enable them to carry out a wide range of functions.

---

7 https://www.researchgate.net/figure/Scheme-of-biological-functions-of-substance-P-Once-the-nerve-ending-catch-noxious_fig12_221917605

Substance P is increased in stressful situations which promote anxiety. Further, stimuli like pain and heat can initiate the release of Substance P from sensory nerve endings which is proportional to the intensity of the stimuli.

It can be seen that as Substance P is associated with inflammatory processes, pain and inflammation can enhance its expression. Such activation appears to become a vicious circle where Substance P is activated by illness or injury and the subsequent pain induces the releases of even more Substance P.

Substance P containing nerves are found in abundance at mucosal sites such as the airway. They are also found in the spinal cord, brain, the skin and around blood vessels. Substance P helps to transmit pain signals to the brain and spinal cord where pain is felt.

Studies have found that a nerve injury can cause a huge release of Substance P which is up to five times greater than in acute pain. It then diffuses out into the local area contributing to persistent pain.

On the other hand, Substance P stimulated the growth of nerve stem cells of adult rats under both normal conditions and during injury. Therefore, it could help with nerve cell formation after injury.

Neuronal substance P is stored in vesicles and released when it comes into contact with
- leukotrienes – which are also involved in the inflammatory response
- prostaglandins
- histamine

among others

Substance P is the main pain messenger in the brain. It has five main functions in the body and these are.

- Pain
- Inflammation
- Anxiety
- Depression
- Nausea

At first glance you wonder why the body is making such a horrible substance but they are important for survival. For example, inflammation is necessary for healing to take place. Pain helps guarding so that we limit movement until it is safe to do otherwise. Problems only occur when there is excessive production and release of it.

Ginger blocks both the production of prostaglandins and leukotrienes as well as Substance P. In cell based studies capsaicin (found in peppers) and curcumin both blocked the production of leukotrienes.

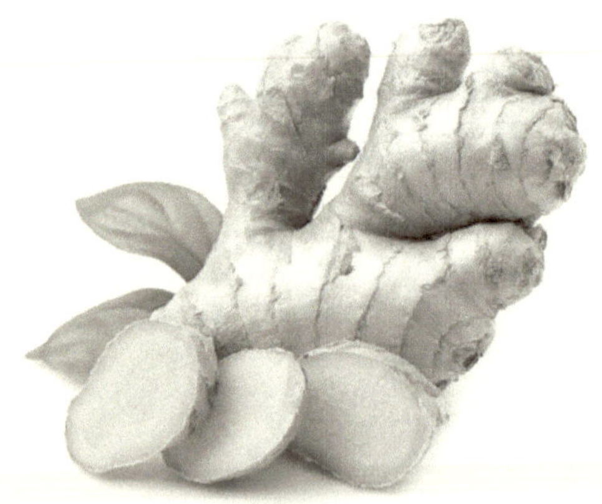

8

The inflammatory processes of Substance P and the subsequent pain can also be addressed by over the counter medications with an anti-inflammatory action like ibuprofen or other NSAID's.

Substance P and rheumatoid arthritis

There are a number of studies which have implicated Substance P in the pain associated with rheumatoid arthritis and other inflammatory disease. There are sensory nerves which release Substance P which are connected to the joint. Further, Substance P was found in higher concentrations in the synovial fluid of patients with rheumatoid arthritis. Finally, there appears to be a greater number of Substance P receptors in rheumatoid tissue.

Lotz[9] et al discovered another possible role for Substance P in arthritis.   It appears that

---

GB828&source=lnms&tbm=isch&sa=X&ved=0ahUKEwix0Kad_cLfAh
WVrHEKHcO4BugQ_AUIDigB&biw=1366&bih=657#imgrc=M6QYox
1dER0mRM:

9

https://www.researchgate.net/publication/282659658_Substance_

Substance P can stimulate synoviocytes (synovial cells) in rheumatoid arthritis. When stimulated the synovial cells increased the release of prostaglandin and collagenase.

Collagenase is an enzyme which breaks down collagen. Collagen is a protein which is found in the bones, skin, muscles, tendons, blood vessel and the digestive organs. Collagen provides the elasticity we find in the skin.

We can take collagen in supplement form which may help build up areas of damaged tissue or we can eat foods which help with collagen formation and these include anything which is skin or bones. Therefore, do not throw away crispy chicken skin. Make bone broth out of bones. It will help keep the wrinkles at bay.

Nevertheless, having done this, the original problem of too much Substance P needs to be addressed first. The inhibitors of Substance P are curcumin, capsaicin and cayenne pepper (which apparently also enhances hair growth).

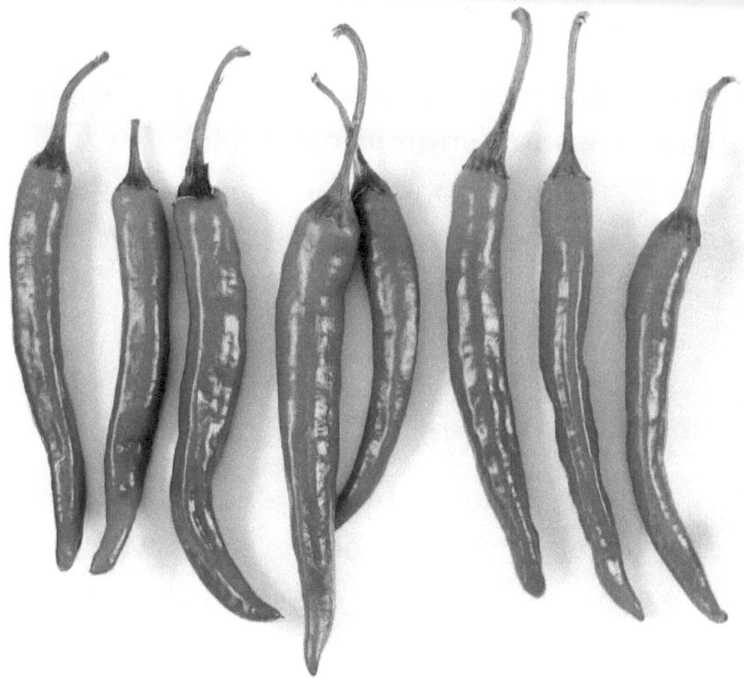

10

Cayenne peppers block Substance P

---

[10] https://www.swansonvitamins.com/blog/lindsey/benefits-of-cayenne-pepper

Other contenders are

Peanut butter

This is rich in magnesium which has an analgesic effect. Magnesium deficiencies encourage the body to make too much Substance P. Peanut butter also contains resveratrol which reduces pain and protects cartilage.

Peanut Curry Sauce

Mix peanut butter with coconut milk, grated, fresh ginger and curry and simmer gently to make a sauce. These type of sauces always taste better when they are made and left in a cool place for the flavours to develop.

Ginger – it is only the fresh ginger root which blocks enzymes which produce inflammatory chemicals.

Use thin sticks of ginger in stir fries or grate a whole ginger root into sparkling water and add honey or other sweetener for home made ginger ale.

Extra Virgin Olive Oil

This contains an anti-inflammatory compound called oleocanthal. This has a similar action to non-steroidal anti inflammatory drugs (NSAID's).

Pineapple

This fruit is rich in an enzyme called bromelain that helps reduce pain and inflammation.

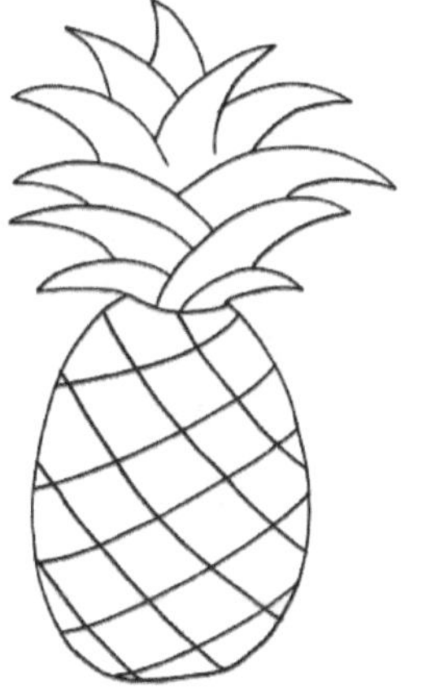

Rheumatoid arthritis and the histamine connection

Histamine is released early on in an inflammatory response and it may be useful to take an antihistamine early on in an acute flare up of this and any other inflammatory condition. It should also be noted that if the diet is low in magnesium then this stimulates the release of histamine from mast cells.

Fibromyalgia and the histamine connection

Fibromyalgia or fibromyalgia syndrome (FMS) is defined by the NHS as

A long term condition that causes pain all over the body. As well as widespread pain, people with fibromyalgia also have increased sensitivity to pain, fatigue (extreme tiredness) and muscle stiffness.

Common problems associated with fibromyalgia are

- Fatigue
- Pain and tender points
- Sleep problems
- Concentration and memory problems
- Headaches
- Anxiety and depression
- Morning stiffness
- Numbness and tingling in the hands, arms, feet and legs.

When we look at the symptoms that histamine can cause, they are not dissimilar. Further, histamine is a substance which causes body wide pain and discomfort. We can discount prostaglandins as being a major player in widespread pain as prostaglandins tend to produce localised pain.

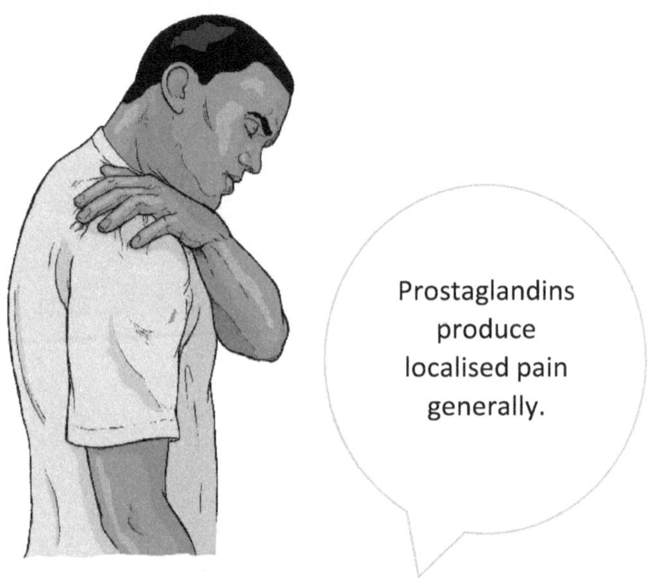

However, prostaglandins could be responsible for the trigger point pain in fibromyalgia.

At this point it would be helpful to tabulate the main inflammatory substances and their characteristics. Having this information to hand can often help you to decide which substance is likely to be producing the pain. In this way, the most likely cause of the pain and the appropriate remedy can be ascertained which will afford the best possible pain relief.

Table showing main inflammatory mediators, mode of action and remedy

Serotonin	Serotonin is a substance which can relieve pain as well as cause it. If it acts in the peripheral nervous system, then it worsens pain in inflammation and nerve injury. Chronic pain causes serotonin to be released by the brain into the spinal cord. Studies show that surrounding uninjured areas appear sensitive to

	pain, a phenomenon which is generally found in chronic pain. To lower levels of serotonin, don't eat foods containing carbohydrates and keep light muted as sunlight helps to increase serotonin levels.
Prostaglandin	These are produced by every tissue in the body but only act locally to injury or illness. They respond to NSAIDS such as ibuprofen as well as fresh ginger.
Bradykinins	Produce localised pain and swelling. They respond to bromelain found in pineapple.
. Substance P	Released from the ends of specific sensory nerves in the CNS and the PNS. It has the potential to produce widespread pain. Found in mucosal sites, skin, around blood vessels, spinal cord and

	brain. Fresh ginger and NSAID's act against it.
Histamine	Systemic action – released from mast cells found in nearby connective tissue. Generally found in acute inflammation BUT histamine intolerance can lead to widespread chronic pain. Use over the counter antihistamines to counteract histamines effects and DAO.

Fibromyalgia has a long history and has been renamed a number of times. It was known as fibrositis but 'itis' means inflammation and it did not appear as though there was any widespread inflammation in this condition.

In 1986 the antidepressants that raised brain levels of serotonin and/or nor-epinephrine was found to be effective in the treatment of fibromyalgia.

These drugs amitriptyline and doxepin were also subsequently found to have potent antihistaminic properties.

Over the counter antihistamines work very well on histamine intolerance and have very few, if any, side effects apart from a tendency to cause drowsiness. Some of the newer antihistamines are less likely to cause drowsiness. One of the unwanted side effects of antihistamines is that they have the potential to cause weight gain. This is thought to be due to the fact that histamine reduces appetite. Therefore, antihistamine can increase it.

A natural antihistamine which does not cause weight gain is vitamin C. Megadoses of up to 2000mg can be taken daily but this can cause diarrhoea in susceptible people. In others it can have a pro-inflammatory action even though it has an anti- inflammatory action in most people. With any medical condition a little trial and error will not go amiss until the right treatment at the right dosage is found.

Of course, the methods we used for reducing histamine in rheumatoid arthritis are just as effective for fibromyalgia.

Histamine has entered more and more foods in the food chain. Tomatoes and pickled foods contain lots of histamine. Fermented foods such as cheese and yogurt also contain histamine.

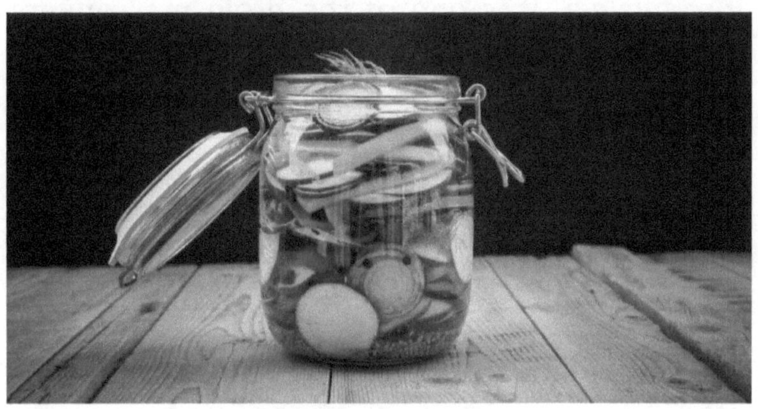

11

Pickled foods contain lots of histamine which can cause widespread pain in susceptible people

[11] http://twistedfood.co.uk/real-reason-communists-absolutely-love-pickled-vegetables/

In 1963 yogurt was introduced by Ski to the UK for the first time. In many cases it has become a daily addition to the diet since it is marketed as being a healthy addition to the diet.

It should be remembered that any food has the potential to be unhealthy for some susceptible people.

Substance P has also been implicated in fibromyalgia. It is one of the brain messengers believed to be dysregulated in fibromyalgia. As it is released from specific sensory nerves found in the central nervous system and the peripheral nervous system, it could account for the specific pain points which sufferers of fibromyalgia have. However, it also causes widespread pain.

The treatment for excessive Substance P is different to that of histamine intolerance and it may be that treatment for both needs to be started together for a couple of weeks. After that, then the treatment for either excessive Substance P or histamine intolerance can be slowly withdrawn to see if it makes a difference.

In any case, when someone has fibromyalgia, a low histamine diet should be considered as it can make a huge difference to an oft misunderstood disease.

In some cases, it may be that the diet is not particularly high in histamine but that the individual does not make enough enzyme called diamine oxidase (DAO). This enzyme deactivates histamine after it has done its job.

Genetics, gastrointestinal issues, such as leaky gut, and some medications can all cause low DAO.

Alison Vickery is a Functional Diagnostic Nutrition Practitioner. In her blog[12] she explains more about DAO and its actions. She states that the intestinal mucosal layer is protective in the gut and contains a wide range of enzymes used in digestion and nutrient absorption. One of these enzymes is DAQ.

Alison goes on to say that DAO protects the body against an excessive build-up of histamines by

____

[12] https://alisonvickery.com.au/category/blog/

degrading histamine which has been eaten and further, bacterial histamine.

Sometimes a genetic mutation reduces the synthesis of DAO in the body. However, we can get it from food.

Protein

Protein is responsible for the release of DAO in the gut. It helps release DAO from the intestinal mucosa into the gut to deal with ingested and bacterial amines and histamines.

Fat

Oleic acid dramatically increases the release of DAO into the bloodstream by up to 500%. Olive oil is one of the primary sources of oleic acid.

Olive oil contains salicylates and can cause an intolerance to those with a susceptibility as such. If this applies to you , then you need to look at alternative ways of increasing DAO or decreasing histamine as outlined in the section on histamine and rheumatoid arthritis.

Canola oil is also a good source of oleic acid but, unfortunately, it is also highly inflammatory. Therefore, I would not advise using this.

Other good sources of DAO are poultry and lamb.

Finally, malic acid which is found in apples and pears has also been found to reduce the pain of fibromyalgia. Some cold pressed juice would not go amiss, in this case.

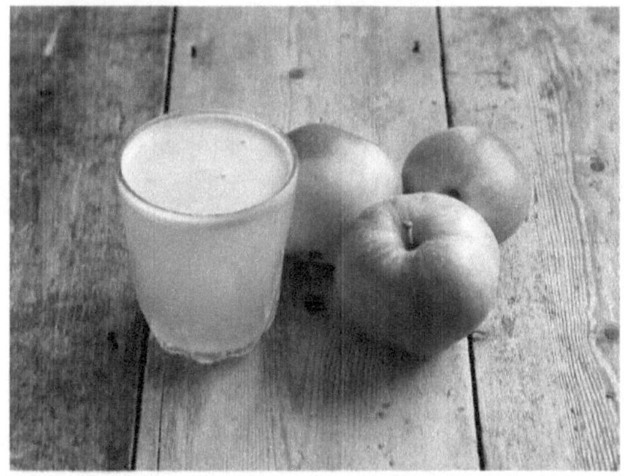

[13] **Malic acid in apples has been found to relieve the pain of fibromyalgia**

[13] https://www.abelandcole.co.uk/apples-for-juicing-5kg?gclid=CjOKCQiAsJfhBRCaARIsAO68ZM56Z7X8NIGgtXdkiq1ou-pldMRiHiSQ3vet_d9XiOK6D7s4Z11rdqwaAi-vEALw_wcB

The pain associated with osteoarthritis

Osteoarthritis is the commonest type of arthritis. About 50% of the population over the age of sixty years will suffer from this condition. It is a condition of older age and is generally, but not always, found in those over fifty years of age.

It is twice as common in women than it is in men and further, it is more prevalent in the white population than the black population.

Osteoarthritis is not considered to be an inflammatory disease. It occurs when the surface of the joint is damaged so that the smooth cartilage is not producing a cushioned surface between the ends of the bones.

The cartilage is normally a shock absorber but can become worn and thin. This means the bone it is meant to protect suffers and becomes thicker. The process is slow and occurs generally in the weight bearing joints such as the hips and knees.

As the bone thickens bony outcrops grow into the joint membranes which usually become inflamed with synovial fluid. This can cause some swelling around the joint.

The main symptoms are pain and stiffness with reduced joint movement.

Due to lack of use which is caused by the pain, muscle mass is lost. One of the major treatments on the NHS is physiotherapy so that muscle tone is built up and the sufferer can continue to exercise. The helps to avoid excessive weight gain which can progress osteoarthritis.

Remedies for the pain for osteoarthritis.

Vitamin B3

This was a popular remedy in the 1930's when the choice of NSAID's wasn't available. In particular, nicotinamide or niacin – both alternative names for vitamin B3 was found to improve grip strength and joint mobility when a particular treatment plan was given. This involved taking 250mg of vitamin B3 every one and a half hours for a daily total of ten doses. That is 2500mg per day.

Nicotinamide is generally given over niacin because the latter causes a warm flush when it is given. Not all people object to this but some do.

Other studies have shown that B6 shrinks the synovial membranes that line the weight bearing surfaces of the joints. Clearly, this helps control pain and restore mobility in the joints such as the hips, knees, shoulders and elbows.

Any B vitamin should be taken in conjunction with the family of B vitamins. One table of the vitamin B complex obtained from the supermarket should be quite sufficient to provide the 75-300mg of pyridoxine required to shrink the synovial membranes.

Vitamin C

Whenever 'itis' occurs at the end of a word, it refers to inflammation. Whenever there is inflammation then vitamin C should be involved in the treatment plan. Vitamin C neutralises the free radicals which damage tissues and reduces inflammation.

Our diets are largely deficient in vitamin C if we eat a lot of processed foods. Vitamin C is easily destroyed by cooking and sunlight. The recommended daily allowance of 30mg hardly seems enough when there are so many inflammatory conditions around

A deficiency of vitamin C produces scurvy and one of the symptoms of scurvy is joint problems. Vitamin C is also required to form collagen which is necessary for healthy joints, bones, ligaments and tendons.

When joint problems do occur, vitamin C can be given in increasing 500mg doses until the tissues are saturated. At this point the beginnings of diarrhoea will occur so you need to lower the dose a little until you find a dose which promotes healing but doesn't produce loose stools. Some people can tolerate much higher levels of vitamin C before it affects their stool in which they can safely take higher doses of vitamin C. Any excess of this vitamin will simply be passed out of the body in urine.

Juniper berries

Sebastian Knapp was a 19th century priest and healer. He often prescribed juniper berries for a number of ailments. Juniper is able to cure rheumatism, skin disorders and gout. A little tipple of sloe gin would not go amiss and I know of a number of people for whom it works well.

Pectin and grape juice

This is another of those recipes which has been tried and tested by many with good results. Pectin and apple residue has been used in regenerative medicine in diseases such as osteoporosis, arthritis or osteoarthritis. Resveratrol found in red grapes has powerful anti-inflammatory effects so the above mix is a good treatment for osteoarthritis.

Certo is a proprietary pectin although you can make your own. We grow seven different varieties of apples and we cannot store 500 apples so we often make pectin from the skins and freeze it. We don't like to waste anything.

Just this afternoon I was talking to a gentleman who told me about the success he had for his arthritic knees after taking a tablespoon of cider vinegar every day.

There is no reason why the above cannot be combined to taste.

I use apples in soup a lot. It is a good base and enhances the flavour of soup. I also add it to casserole meats when they are cooking in the slow cooker, they thicken the gravy and produce a delicious gravy. There really aren't many dishes that you can't add apples to. They really are versatile. It is easy to see why the saying 'an apple a day keeps the doctor away' was coined.

Bone broths

I cannot praise enough the contribution of bone broths to the prevention and repair of cartilage.

Cartilage is difficult to repair as it has a poor blood supply but we have also thrown a lot of our healing foods away as society has 'advanced.'

One of these habits that we have dispensed with is boiling the bones up off joints of meat. This takes long slow cooking and most people consider that they don't have time nowadays or realise just how delicious and healthy it is.

If I have a chicken, then I keep the carcase and throw it into the slow cooker with some onions and some apple peelings (I keep these in the freezer for such a time as this). I eventually strain the stock which can be used for soups stews or risottos. It is delicate and delicious and is one of the best medicines you can have for your joints. I generally add some lemon juice to the water the bones simmer in as it helps the bones soften and the nutrients come out.

If you add this stock to a curry, then there are added anti-inflammatory benefits with the curcumin but really the beauty of bone broth is the gelatine which helps build up cartilage.

Manganese is a mineral which is necessary for the enzymatic synthesis of an enzyme called mucopolysaccharide which has been found to be deficient in people with rheumatoid arthritis.

Mucopolysaccharide is as substance which help to cushion the joint. It makes the synovial fluid thick and stretchy. This is necessary if the joints are not to become damaged as thin, watery fluid cannot cushion the joints properly. This means that the cartilage and bone will scrape against each other and, of course, this means that the cartilage erodes.

Research has shown that adequate levels of manganese is essential to the synthesis of mucopolysaccharide. There is also some evidence that an adequate intake of manganese could also repair cartilage.

Manganese is found in:

- Nuts, such as almonds
- Beans and legumes
- Whole cereals
- Green leafy vegetables

- Dark chocolate
- Pineapple
- Egg yolks
- Sunflower seeds

Copper – when the causes of rheumatoid arthritis are considered, people generally think of it in terms of:

- The body being unable to produce enough antibodies to fight off viruses which are damaging the joints
- The antibodies which are being produced are unable to distinguish which is a foreign body and which is your own tissue so it attacks self
- Allergies sometimes cause rheumatoid arthritis.

However, copper also plays a part. Copper is a component of an antioxidant enzyme called Superoxidase Dismutase (SOD). SOD is able to prevent damage to the membrane and synovial fluid of the joints.

It appears that copper interacts with pigments in fats to inhibit free radical formation which has damaging effects on the joints and surrounding structures.

Copper does not necessarily need supplementing in food as it is so widely available in the diet. It can be found in:

- Wholegrain foods
- Meat
- Raisins
- legumes

MSM

Methylsulfonylmethane is another compound which has numerous benefits for relieving pain although stiffness does not appear to respond as well. It is found in many fruits and vegetables but can also be obtained from health food stores as a powder which can be sprinkled over food.

Phenylalanine

This is an essential amino acid which has excellent pain relieving properties regardless of the cause of the pain. It is an adjunctive substance which means it can be used alongside your regular pain control and will enhance the pain relieving effect.

It can be bought at any health food store as a powder. It has a slight taste which is not unpleasant and can be taken with water although it does not mix well.

Chondroitin Sulphate

Supplements for chondroitin sulfate generally come from animal cartilage. A study found that glucosamine and chondroitin were as effective for knee osteoarthritis as a well- known NSAID. It is claimed to reduce pain and inflammation and improves joint cartilage.

Magnesium is an effective pain relief mineral and also inhibits the breakdown of cartilage. Most people are magnesium deficient anyway. There is more likely to be a deficiency if the individual is using diuretics or laxatives.

Tendonitis

Tendons can be found wherever a muscle needs to be connected to a bone knees, shoulders and elbows are well known one.

It is generally a condition of overuse and depending where it is located or how it was caused can be described as such. Therefore, we have terms such as golfer's elbow or tennis elbow.

Tendonitis frequently occurs in those with hypermobile joints. That is the joints extend beyond the normal range. Sometimes people will refer to themselves as double jointed. Their knee joints may bend backwards too much, for example or they may be able to touch their wrist with their thumb on the same side. These are examples of hypermobile joints. (see overleaf).

Hypermobile knees

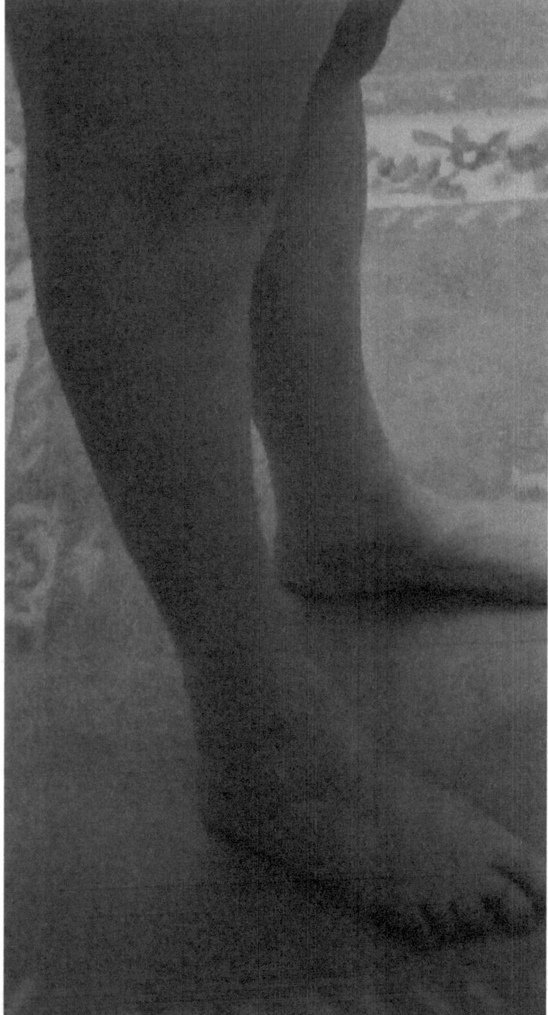

Note the curvature of these hypermobile joints

When joints are hypermobile, then it is better to splint them, or provide some support, if being involved in heavy exercise.

The main symptoms of tendonitis are:

- Pain in a tendon which gets worse when you use it
- A lump along the tendon
- Swelling with heat and redness
- Feeling a grating or crackling sensation when you move the tendon

Tendonitis can sometimes take a long time to heal. In the initial acute inflammatory stages, tendonitis can render a joint virtually useless with the pain. It does eventually resolve but it can take so long that the sufferer fears that it will never go.

If it lasts longer than 6 months, then you could ask for a referral to see the physiotherapist. Rest is essential but the sufferer will not take much persuading that this is the best course of action.

As tendonitis is an inflammatory condition then the methods used for conditions which have already been discussed for inflammation and pain relief will suffice.

Alternating warmth and cold packs for twenty minutes generally helps healing but it must be emphasised that in the initial few days after injury, or a flare up of an inflammatory disorder, that only cold packs should be used.

The reasoning behind this is that inflammation produces heat. We do not require any more heat as this will just increase the pain. Shortly after an injury there are likely to be many tiny blood vessels which have ruptured and are bleeding into the tissue surrounding it. This is how a bruise is formed. It is painful because there is increased fluid and other substances pressing on the nerves around the injury. Applying heat will cause the blood vessels to open up and bleed further into the area around the injury. This is what we do not want. Therefore, the application of cold is recommended only for three days before alternating cold and heat can be considered. If the area is still hot and red, continue with the application of cold only.

Similarly, after any injury NSAID's such as ibuprofen should never be taken for the first two days. This is entirely due to the effects of anti-inflammatories which thin the blood and promote bleeding into the injured tissue. This is why athletes bathe in very cold water after an important race. The effect of such exertion will cause tiny tears in muscle tissue which bleed and cause pain. Bathing in cold water will reduce this phenomenon and any associated pain. If pain relief is required, then paracetamol is the best choice of painkiller for this type of injury in the early days.

The acronym rice, often quoted, needs to be applied just as often.

Rest

Ice

Compression

Elevation

Bursitis

A bursa is a fluid filled sac which forms under the skin usually over joints. It acts as a cushion between the tendons and the bones. Bursitis is inflammation and swelling of the bursa. This causes pain and tenderness at the site of the injury.

The most common areas which are affected by bursitis are the

- Knee (also known as housemaid's knee)
- Shoulder
- Elbow
- Hip

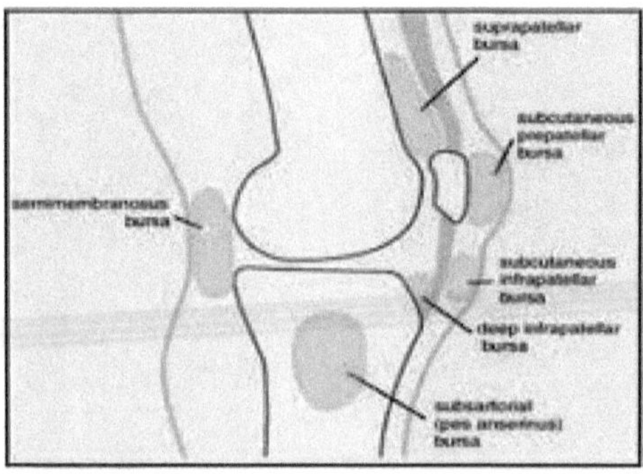

Bursitis is caused by injury and repetitive movement. Shoulder bursitis can occur in those who play badminton regularly. Darts players can develop bursitis of the elbow. Gardeners tend to develop housemaid's knee since they – and floor layers – spend a lot of time on their knees.

Bursitis, however, can also develop as a result of an infection or as a complication of certain conditions such as rheumatoid arthritis. Rheumatoid arthritis affects the synovial capsule which encapsulates the joint.

Any condition ending in 'itis' is an inflammatory condition and, as such, responds to vitamin C and ice. I generally use a bag of frozen peas in a tea towel. If the bursitis is due to an injury, keep off the ibuprofen for a couple of days and substitute paracetamol instead. After a couple of days, ibuprofen and paracetamol may be taken together. They are far more effective this way. They should be taken for as little time as is possible. Ibuprofen can damage the stomach lining so should always be taken after eating. This is because prostaglandins actually help protect the lining of the stomach from acid which can eat away at the stomach and produce an ulcer. NSAID's, of course, reduce the production of prostaglandins which cause stomach irritation.

Prostaglandins also aid in removal of fluid via the kidneys so that fluid retention will be one side effect of taking NSAID's. They also interfere with platelet function and possibly increase the risk of bleeding and clotting time.

Prostaglandins are synthesised in the body from poly unsaturated fatty acids (PUFA's). Most people do not know that the oils that we use in cooking nowadays such as sunflower oil and rape seed oil have an inflammatory action. The rise in inflammatory joint problems may partially be as a result of us exchanging the saturated fats that we used to use in cooking (lard, dripping and butter) for these apparently healthy cooking oils.

Further, ibuprofen has been shown, in studies, to wipe out the first 0-4 days of the acute inflammatory response. While we do not enjoy the pain and discomfort that the inflammatory response brings, it is essential for healing. The only time we should be concerned is if continues for a long time and becomes 'chronic' pain. Chronic pain is that which occurs for more than twelve weeks. [14]

Paracetamol's pain killing actions occur in the central nervous system and ibuprofen's in the peripheral nervous system.

It does take a while for the pain to go permanently. The swelling will take slightly longer. It should go without saying that any activity that has caused the bursitis in the first place, should cease until the injury has healed. If an infection is present, then the GP may prescribe antibiotics.[15]

It is easy to lose muscle mass when a limb has to be rested. Gentle exercise is often recommended by a physiotherapist until healing has taken place and patience is the key.

---

[14] The subject of acute and chronic pain is addressed in Pain: its causes and responses.
[15] Treat Infection Naturally by Lynne D M Noble

Boron

Boron is a trace mineral or micronutrient with diverse and essential roles in metabolism. It is essential for the growth and maintenance of bone, greatly improves wound healing and impacts on how the body uses oestrogen, testosterone and vitamin D. Further, it boosts magnesium absorption and reduces levels of inflammatory biomarkers such as C-reactive protein and tumour necrosis factor.

Boron[16] has also been found to raise levels of important antioxidants such as superoxide (SOD), catalase and glutathione peroxidase.

In recent human trials, a significant increase in concentrations of plasma boron occurred 6 hours after supplementation with 11.6mg of boron coupled with significant decreases – of 20% - in TNF when 10mg daily was taken for a week and further, a 50% decrease of the inflammatory marker hs-CRP.

---

[16] https://www.ncbi.nlm.nih.gov/pmc/articles/PMC4712861/

Boron improves bone and joint health too. The recommendation is 3mg a day if the diet is low in fruit and vegetables. These can be sourced online or at a health food shop. Boron can be found in:

- Apples
- Almonds
- Chickpeas
- Beans
- bananas

GABA – neuropathic pain is pain that results from a malfunction in the nervous system. Sometimes, neuropathic pain occurs alongside inflammatory disorders and in auto-immune conditions such as rheumatoid arthritis.

Neuropathic pain does not go away after the stimulus which initiated it ends. Neuropathic pain can feel 'weird.' For example, pain results from a light touch and have sufferers often have an inability to be able to regulate their body temperature.

GABA is a signalling chemical and is found in spinal nerve cells. These GABA neurons act as a brake on pain impulses.

GABA appears to be particularly sensitive to oxidative stress which may contribute to the loss of these special neurons after tissue damage.

In a study, mice which had been surgically altered to feel neuropathic pain. After being given an antioxidant compound, they were compared with untreated mice who weren't given an antioxidant compound. The treated mice showed less pain behaviour and were found to have more GABA neurons. From this study it appears that antioxidants have therapeutic potential for pain.

The *gate control theory of pain* asserts that non-painful stimuli close the nerve gates to painful input. This prevents the sensation of pain from traveling to the central nervous system. This is the basis on which a TENS machine works. It provides a different non-pain sensation which blocks or suppresses pain.

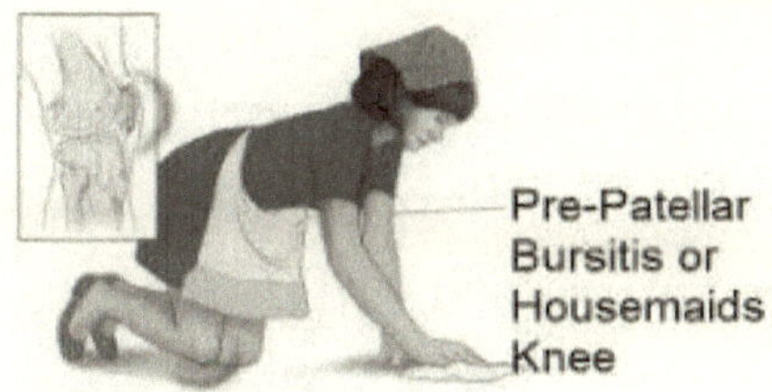

17

---

[17] https://www.wildermanphysicaltherapy.com/is-knee-pain-slowing-you-down-it-just-may-be-bursitis/

The anti-inflammatory diet

There are a great many foods which promote inflammation. It may surprise you that vegetable oils and margarine promote inflammation. They contain omega 6 which is pro-inflammatory. Our diet now contains far more pro-inflammatory foods since the introduction of the above. They are added to many ready foods and used liberally in the home.

Omega 6 should be balanced by the omega 3's. The latter is found in only a limited range of foods such as oily fish and so balancing these is quite difficult.

 The vegetable oils which are the main offenders are sunflower and rapeseed oil (but not olive oil). They promote inflammatory responses in your body. Inflammation is exceedingly aging if it is not legitimately being used to heal an injury or illness.

On the other hands solid fats such as lard, dripping and butter do not promote inflammation. They are relatively stable compared to vegetable oils. They have a high smoking point so do not readily produce free radicals which damage cells.

Fruit and vegetables are anti-inflammatory so these can be eaten freely.

Sugary foods and burnt foods also promote inflammation so these are better kept to a minimum when you have an inflammatory condition.

Other than changing your choice of oils and fats, not charring food, eating fruit and vegetables and reducing the sugar in your diet you can pretty well eat what you normally eat. It will make a difference and the inflammation will die down and eventually disappear.

My husband was eating pork pie and mushy peas the other day. An adjacent diner referred to it as an unhealthy meal due to the fat content. However, the fats used in this dish were the healthy saturated fats. The meal is unlikely to raise blood sugar levels a great deal and it also contains fibre and a good amount of the fat soluble vitamins. It was, indeed, a healthy meal.

The Mediterranean diet incorporates a lot of the above but it differs in that it recommends canola oil as well as olive oil. Canola oil is also referred to as rapeseed oil. Using canola oil is not a wise move due to its highly inflammatory nature (and butter tastes better).

Of course you can use butter to make a salad dressing by slowly melting the butter on a very low heat, throwing some grated lemon peel and herbs or coriander in with it. Let it cool, but not solidify, before tossing the salad into it. We use this a lot and we far prefer it to salad dressing made with oil. However, olive oil does have good anti-inflammatory properties and can be used freely especially if a histamine intolerance is responsible for pain .

Final Thoughts

This book was written with the intention of empowering people to take control over their own pain. Joint and connective tissue pain has the potential to reduce the quality of life greatly but there is a great deal which can be done to alleviate the pain of joint and rheumatic pain.

Traditional medicine does not use all the tools to hand when treating a disease process. For example, they do not provide copper bracelets which many sufferers of arthritis swear by.

Most people do not know of the benefits of enough manganese in the diet or that GABA is very effective at treating pain,

Once you have read this book, it may be useful to go back over it more slowly and build up your own treatment strategy for your own particular medical condition. This is bespoke medicine and you will find what not only controls the pain but what foods you need to eat (or avoid) to reduce or reverse the disease process.

I hope that you have found the answers you are
seeking within.

List of Essential Macro-minerals

- calcium
- chloride
- potassium
- sodium
- magnesium
- sulphur
- phosphorus

List of Essential Micronutrients

- cobalt
- iron
- chromium
- iodine
- zinc
- fluorine
- selenium
- manganese
- copper
- molybdenum
- boron

Thank you for purchasing this book. Every time a book is purchased, a donation is made to one of the charities I am currently supporting. These can be found on my author's website. See below.

Other Health Related Books by the Author

- **The Reluctant Bowel**
- **A Weighty Issue**
- **Sleep, Perchance to Dream**
- **The Journey: EDS and chronic pain**
- **The MND diet: using nutrition to slow down the progress of neurodegeneration**
- **A Necessary Sorrow**
- **Treat infection Naturally**
- **Successful Aging**
- **Taking another Road: Pain: its causes and what can be done about it**
- **Osteoarthritis and Pain**
- **A Treatment Strategy for Migraine**

These can be found here on the author's page

https://www.amazon.co.uk/-/e/B07BPQZ5CD

You may also be interested in the semi-autobiographical trilogy of the authors life found in these three books

- The Prejudged
- Where the Blackbird Never Sings
- A Summer's Symphony

And the author's children's books

- Fanny and Victorian Jack
- Fanny and the Gamekeeper's Cottage